DYSPRAXIA / DCD
Pocketbook

By Afroza Talukdar

Cartoons:
Phil Hailstone

Published by:

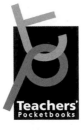

Teachers' Pocketbooks
Laurel House, Station Approach,
Alresford, Hampshire SO24 9JH, UK
Tel: +44 (0)1962 735573
Fax: +44 (0)1962 733637
Email: sales@teacherspocketbooks.co.uk
Website: www.teacherspocketbooks.co.uk

*Teachers' Pocketbooks is an imprint of
Management Pocketbooks Ltd.*

With thanks to Brin Best for his help in
launching the series.

© Afroza Talukdar 2012

This edition published 2012. Reprinted 2015.

ISBN 978 1 906610 38 8

E-book ISBN 978 1 9082 8486 0

British Library Cataloguing-in-Publication
Data – A catalogue record for this book is
available from the British Library.

Design, typesetting and graphics by Efex Ltd.
Printed in UK.

Contents

Foreword

Since the turn of the 21st century, the scientific and medical literature has been peppered with case reports of children without an identifiable medical or neurological condition, who appeared physically and intellectually normal, yet who lacked the movement competence necessary to cope with the demands of everyday living. These children had previously been described by parents, teachers and peers as 'clumsy' children. The condition is now widely referred to as 'dyspraxia' or 'Developmental Co-ordination Disorder' (DCD).

Although children with dyspraxia/DCD have always been in schools, the formal identification of motor (ie movement) skills is a fairly recent phenomenon. There has been a marked increase in the number of children with developmental co-ordination disorder in the last 20 years but considerable uncertainty still exists around its accurate diagnosis because of its co-existence with other disorders, such as dyslexia, dyscalculia, dysgraphia, ADHD, autistic spectrum disorders and specific language difficulties.

In some situations it can be hard to identify the principal difficulty or difficulties experienced by the child.

Foreword

In this Pocketbook, I hope to provide a better understanding and insight into the 'hidden disability' of dyspraxia/DCD. The book explains how dyspraxia/DCD can affect an individual and outlines the challenges they might face. It focuses on how to support children to learn to cope with the demands of the classroom environment and to allow them maximal learning opportunities and participation. The book also describes the common characteristics of children with motor co-ordination difficulties and provides guidance on early identification and interventions so that a pupil's self-esteem and positive social interactions with peers can be enhanced.

Foreword

Specialist and non-specialist teachers as well as parents and teaching assistants in both primary and secondary schools will find this book useful. It includes practical strategies that will allow the full potential of every learner with dyspraxia/DCD to be unlocked in the classroom.

However, each person with dyspraxia/DCD is unique, which means that each has their own set of strengths and difficulties. As a result, when reading this book please bear in mind that some strategies will be more appropriate for some children than others.

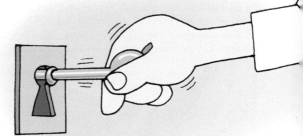

What is Dyspraxia/DCD?

Dypraxia or DCD?

Understanding dyspraxia/ DCD can be very confusing because so many terms have been used to describe the condition. Both nationally and internationally, there continues to be a lack of consensus regarding both the definition and description of this disorder.

The terms most often used today are 'dyspraxia' or 'developmental co-ordination disorder' (DCD).

DCD is an umbrella term encompassing dyspraxia. Strictly speaking, dyspraxia is a more specific example of DCD and is a more sensory-based difficulty, whilst developmental co-ordination disorder is a more motor-based difficulty. In practice, the distinction is rarely made and the two are often merged by professionals and parents. 'Dyspraxia' is recognised by the majority of people as the generic term to explain a range of movement difficulties.

Other terminology

The box below lists the myriad terms used to describe children with movement difficulties who would now be given a diagnosis of dyspraxia or developmental co-ordination disorder.

Other terminology used to describe the condition

- Developmental apraxia
- Perceptual motor-difficulties
- Physically awkward, poorly co-ordinated
- Motor-learning disorder/difficulties
- Deficit in attention, motor and perception (DAMP)
- Neuro-developmental difficulties/dysfunction
- Sensory integrative dysfunction
- Non-verbal learning difficulty
- Minimal cerebral palsy
- Developmental dyspraxia

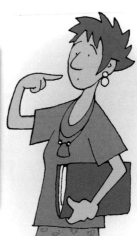

Defining dyspraxia

'Dyspraxia' is derived from the Greek word 'dys', meaning faulty/poor and 'praxis' meaning doing/use of the body. It is best described as a motor learning difficulty, characterised by impairment in the ability to plan and carry out sensory and motor tasks. The main difference between dyspraxia and DCD is that pupils with dyspraxia do not know what to do because they have difficulty making sense of the different messages coming to the brain from their sensory organs. In comparison, pupils with DCD know what they want to do but have difficulty telling their muscles how to move.

A lack of agreement about dyspraxia and DCD difficulties leads to differences in diagnostic accuracy between different medical professionals working with the condition and, consequently, the medical approaches to assessment and treatment also vary.

The Dyspraxia Foundation (1998) defines dyspraxia as *'an impairment or immaturity of the organisation of movement. Associated with this there may be problems of language, perception and thoughts.'*

For the purposes of this book, I will be referring to the condition as 'dyspraxia', whilst acknowledging that, in fact, there is a subtle difference between dyspraxia and DCD.

What we know

Here's what we know about dyspraxia:

- The term 'dyspraxia' is used to explain a range of movement difficulties in the absence of problems with the muscles themselves
- It is a medical diagnosis but there are no blood tests or scans to diagnose it
- It is not a single disease but it is a collection of symptoms
- It is not linked to a pupil's age or intellect
- It is present from birth but becomes more apparent as the child gets older
- It is a life-long condition but it is not a progressive or life-threatening illness
- It can be mild or severe and can affect each person in different ways
- Not all pupils with the diagnosis display the same difficulties
- It is a hidden problem – pupils with dyspraxia look the same as their peers but have real difficulty with movement activities, such as riding a bike
- Dyspraxia has a profound impact on a pupil's self-esteem and confidence

What causes dyspraxia?

We know that in people with dyspraxia there is *'an immaturity in the way that the brain processes information, which results in messages not being properly or fully transmitted'**. What we do not know is what causes this.

There is no evidence to suggest clinical neurological abnormality in people with dyspraxia. The prevailing view is that the causes are likely to be genetic in basis with interaction with the environment, eg prematurity, increasing the risk. Further research is needed.

*Dyspraxia Foundation - www.dyspraxiafoundation.org.uk

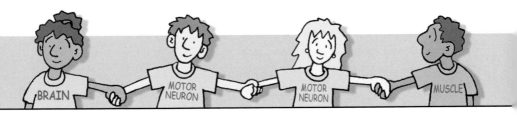

How common is dyspraxia?

Research has shown that, on average, around 6% of pupils have some degree of dyspraxia; some authors consider the figure to be as high as 10%. A true figure is difficult to obtain as dyspraxia commonly occurs with other conditions (more later).

It's reasonable to assume that at least one pupil in an average class of 30 will have motor co-ordination difficulties. Boys are four times more likely to be affected than girls.

As all aspects of development are linked, the movement difficulty (even when it appears to be subtle) has a significant impact on a pupil's subsequent social, emotional and intellectual development and may impair the pupil's normal process of learning.

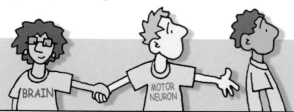

Can dyspraxia be cured?

There is no 'cure' for dyspraxia but, like other specific learning difficulties, if it is identified at an early stage much can be done to mitigate its effect on a pupil's learning and emotional wellbeing.

Most interventions aim to develop the motor skills of pupils with dyspraxia. The evidence suggests that if an effective motor-based programme is implemented regularly, it not only improves a pupil's motor performance but also has a positive impact on their attention and concentration.

Although these difficulties do not ever simply 'go away', early identification and appropriate interventions may allow pupils to develop various coping strategies, build confidence and self-esteem and make good progress in all areas.

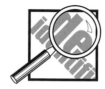

Approaches to Identification

Medical diagnosis and co-existence with other conditions

Dyspraxia is a recognised medical diagnosis. It is based on specific DSM IV (*Diagnostic and Statistical Manual IV*) and ICD 10 criteria (*International Classification of Diseases, 10th Revision*) with no specific cut-off point to determine who has or does not have the condition; rather, it is based on the functional difficulties of the pupil.

Dyspraxia rarely exists in isolation and over half of children with the condition will have also been diagnosed with other conditions such as ADHD or ASD. Dyspraxia can also commonly co-exist with specific language impairments or with specific learning difficulties such as dyslexia, dyscalculia and dysgraphia.

Degree of overlap with other specific learning difficulties

Think of dyspraxia as one of a family of similar conditions, along with ADHD, dyslexia, and autism that arise due to problems with early brain development.

Having any one of these conditions puts pupils at higher risk of having another condition at the same time – we call this an overlap. No two pupils will have the same degree of overlap; one pupil may have dyspraxia, with overlap of dyslexia and dysgraphia; one may have dyspraxia with ADHD; and another, dyspraxia with ASD and ADHD, etc

It is important to recognise and address any other specific learning difficulties that the learner also has, as well as their dyspraxia.

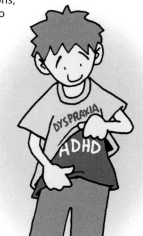

Overlap

How dyspraxia can overlap with other SpLD

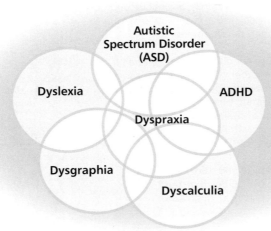

Making the right diagnosis

Diagnosing dyspraxia accurately can be quite difficult in practice. As we have seen, 'dyspraxia' can have different meanings to different professionals and can co-exist with a number of other learning difficulties.

Physiotherapists, occupational therapists, speech and language therapists and paediatricians may all use different descriptions and labels for a pupil's difficulty and therefore the final diagnosis may depend on which professionals have seen and assessed a pupil first. In addition, some specific learning difficulties, such as ADHD and ASD, are medical diagnoses and need to be made by health professionals, whilst others, such as dyslexia, are not.

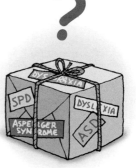

For example, if a pupil is seen by an occupational therapist or a paediatrician, they may be given the primary diagnosis of dyspraxia or DCD. If the same pupil is seen by a clinical psychologist, they may get a primary diagnosis of Asperger syndrome, or ASD, and the speech and language therapist may give a diagnosis of semantic pragmatic disorder (see page 26), which is all extremely confusing!

Individual strengths and weaknesses

Each pupil with dyspraxia will have a unique combination of difficulties, broadly classified into the areas of **motor**, **social**, **language** and **perception**, which can affect many aspects of their life.

Pupils with dyspraxia are unlikely to have problems in all areas. The pattern of difficulty varies widely from person to person and it is important to understand that a major weakness for one pupil with a diagnosis of dyspraxia can be a strength for another, eg some pupils with dyspraxia may have difficulty with reading and spelling due to an overlap with dyslexia, whilst others may be strong readers and spellers.

The key thing is to understand that all pupils are different and will have unique combinations of strengths and weaknesses; it is important to acknowledge what a pupil *can* do as well as what they cannot.

Dyspraxia as a continuum

As with any other specific learning difficulty there is a continuum of need for pupils with dyspraxia. The condition can affect pupils of all abilities and the severity of their impairments will vary from mild to severe.

Pupils may have different cognitive and emotional profiles, strengths, weaknesses and learning preferences.

Some may experience difficulties in several areas; others may have problems in only one.

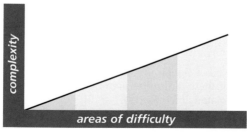

Specific language impairment

Where pupils with a diagnosis of dyspraxia have overlapping language impairments, their speech may be immature, unintelligible or delayed. Some may have good expressive language but have difficulty in social communication skills and understanding (receptive language difficulty).

Examples of language difficulties include:

- Limited vocabulary
- Word finding difficulties
- Poor language concepts and comprehension
- Problem in interpreting, processing and following verbal information
- Literal understanding and difficulty in 'reading between the lines'
- Hesitant or sloppy speech

Language impairment often has a significant impact, not only on a pupil's learning but also on their social life. If these difficulties are not identified and addressed, the pupil can become socially isolated and unhappy.

Supporting children with co-existing language impairment

It is important to identify the nature of a pupil's language difficulty. A pupil with unclear speech is relatively easy to identify, however *receptive* language difficulties may present more subtly. Pupils with receptive language difficulty tend to struggle with:

- Language concepts, eg prepositions such as 'next to', 'above', 'behind', 'under'
- Organising and sequencing ideas and thoughts
- Time concepts, eg 'yesterday', 'a long time ago'
- Mathematical language, eg long/short, big/small

If you have identified a pupil with difficulties in this area, talk to your school's SEN co-ordinator/ inclusion manager about referral to a speech and language therapist for further assessment, specialist advice and interventions.

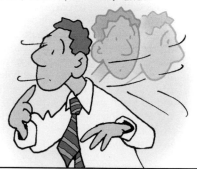

Supporting pupils with co-existing language impairment

Understanding abstract concepts, like 'fairness' or 'freedom', and emotions such as 'love' are much harder for children with language impairments, as these concepts have different meanings in different contexts. For younger children, the concept of 'fair' may mean sharing toys equally and for older pupils, it may mean how you deal with a particular issue in a particular situation.

Pupils with dyspraxia need opportunities to practise and generalise conceptual language in different contexts. Use a multi-sensory approach and use visual aids, eg pictures, real objects, charts, graphs, to teach new concepts and vocabulary. Provide visual links to map new information to previously learned knowledge and to teach subject-specific concepts, for instance using mind or concept maps for teaching 'the water cycle'. Venn diagrams are also useful visual teaching aids.

Verbal dyspraxia

Some pupils have a diagnosis of 'verbal dyspraxia' as well as generalised dyspraxia, which means they have difficulty in making and co-ordinating movements of the speech muscles in their mouth to make clear speech. They have difficulty in producing individual sounds as well as in co-ordinating the sequence of sounds necessary for making words and sentences. They are often unable to communicate under pressure which leads to frustration. Most of these pupils require advice and support from a speech and language therapist to develop their communication skills.

In the classroom, to increase their participation, both verbally and non-verbally, provide:

- Opportunities for role play, drama, group games, and turn-taking activities, where pupils are encouraged to communicate informally and spontaneously

- 'Low-pressure' non-verbal tasks/activities, eg adult-led language games/activities, where pupils are encouraged to participate without feeling pressured to communicate verbally, instead relying on gestures or actions

Semantic pragmatic disorder

A vast proportion of our communication is non-verbal, using body language such as eye contact, hand gestures, body stance, etc. Some pupils with dyspraxia have difficulty in understanding and using verbal and non-verbal language appropriately in different social situations. They find it hard to understand complex social cues such as social distance and etiquette. Speech and language therapists call this 'semantic pragmatic disorder'.

Pupils may also have difficulty in modulating their speech/language/voice/volume/tone with different people in different contexts and as a result they become socially isolated.

To give an example, they may use formal language and voice in all contexts, which might be seen as 'odd' by their peers. Their understanding will also be very literal, so if you say *'keep your chin up'*, they will do just that. You need to provide safe contexts and real-life examples to teach and practise different gestures, emotions and other non-verbal social cues, eg that shrugging shoulders means 'don't know', etc.

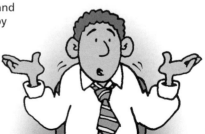

What is
Dyspraxia/DCD?

 Approaches to
Identification

 Effects and
Classroom
Strategies

 Perceptual
Function

 Secondary
Consequences

 Problems with
Motor Memory

 Learning New
Skills

 Developing a
Dyspraxia-friendly
Classroom

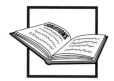

Effects and Classroom Strategies

How can I recognise a pupil with dyspraxia?

A pupil with dyspraxia may:

- Appear clumsy or awkward in their movements. They may frequently bump into objects, trip over, spill and knock things over
- Have difficulties with fine and gross motor activities, such as writing, ball skills
- Have good intellectual and verbal skills but have poor motor performance
- Struggle with daily living activities, such as brushing teeth, tying shoelaces
- Avoid or appear to be uninterested in physical activities
- Exhibit secondary emotional problems, such as low self-esteem, lack of motivation, loneliness and behaviour difficulties
- Have poor organisational skills

The good news is that you can help them by identifying their educational and emotional needs and their strengths and weaknesses. You can also work with them to boost their self-esteem and confidence. Discuss all these areas with them, so that they understand the way they learn best. Most pupils with dyspraxia respond well to multi-sensory approaches; others may have a preferred alternative learning style.

Main areas of difficulties

Learners with dyspraxia are a heterogeneous group. As we have seen, each has a unique combination of difficulties which can affect many aspects of their life.

The most common areas of difficulties are:

- **Cognitive** – difficulties with reading, writing, spelling, short term memory, attention and concentration
- **Speech** – articulation, understanding, processing, sequencing and organising ideas
- **Physical** – problems with balance, co-ordination, gross and fine motor skills
- **Perception** – problems with sensory integration, auditory and visual perception, hypo/hypersensitivity, spatial awareness, orientation and organisation
- **Behaviour** – fidgety, distractibility, immaturity, extreme emotions, low self-esteem
- **Social** – difficulties with social interactions, unable to develop and maintain friendships, may be seen as a 'loner', withdrawn
- **Psychological difficulties** – poor self-confidence, self-esteem, lack of motivation, bullying. They may show anxiety, frustration, anger and jealousy

Discrepancy in intellectual and movement competence

A learner with dyspraxia often has average or above-average intelligence but their performance in activities involving motor co-ordination is substantially below their verbal performance.

Despite their intelligence, they are unable to carry out motor tasks such as playing football with their peers. They may also have difficulty with creative writing, which requires the sequencing of ideas and thoughts, leaving them feeling frustrated. They cannot understand why they are unable to perform physical tasks like their peers and start to see themselves as failures and lose their motivation, self-esteem and confidence. This has a very significant impact on their social, emotional and cognitive development. As they get older, more negative feelings start to grow.

With early interventions and strategies, pupils develop good coping strategies and are more likely to experience success, socially and academically.

Intelligence average or above average

Frustration gap

Motor performance below average

Focus on 'whole pupil' not just the label

A label of 'dyspraxia' does not provide a full explanation of the difficulties within a learner. Each learner will view their difficulties in a unique way and it is vital to understand a pupil's insight as well as parental perspectives. For example, imagine you have identified two boys with dyspraxia. Exploring the background of one of them, you find that his brother has just been selected to play for the school's football team; exploring the background of the other, you find he is frustrated because his friends invite him to play football with them every lunchtime but he is unable to join in, leaving him socially isolated. Only by analysing and assessing the 'whole pupil' and seeing their difficulties in context can you provide strategies for success and optimum learning conditions. A useful approach with the first pupil would be to identify a different strength that he can showcase. For the other boy, a good strategy would be to find alternative group activities that the friends can all participate in.

Many people with dyspraxia also have a spectrum of difficulties with cognitive process that influence attention and concentration, time management, short-term memory and organisational skills. The rest of this section will cover these four areas and suggest intervention strategies to address these difficulties.

Difficulty with short-term memory

Learners with dyspraxia have problems with their short-term memory. This commonly becomes apparent in the classroom when the student has difficulty following instructions. They may not be able to remember everything that you have asked them to do, perhaps only retaining the first or last part of the instruction. So, if you tell the pupil, *'Get your maths book out and write the date and title at the top of the page with a pencil'*, they might manage just to get their pencil out, whilst forgetting the rest. Their difficulty in following instructions is due to:

- **Slow verbal information processing skills** – they take too long to process one aspect of the instruction and are therefore unable to access/ process the rest

- **Auditory sequential memory difficulty** – they have a problem in remembering the sequence of verbal instructions

Short-term memory difficulties may also lead to difficulties sustaining sufficient concentration to perform mental operations, and often reasoning and comprehension skills do not develop appropriately.

Reducing memory overload

It is important to reduce short-term memory overload to sustain the learner's attention and concentration. Routine and structure help pupils to store information in long-term memory – they support the development of 'time awareness' and the ability to carry out tasks more quickly.

Reducing verbal information will minimise processing demands and memory overload:

- Provide short, simple instructions with visual support/ visual reminders of key points
- Deliver instructions slowly and clearly, so that learners have time to process
- Encourage pupils to verbalise instructions, which helps them to understand and store the information in their working memory. If necessary, students could be asked to repeat instructions back to you in their own words
- Gain a learner's attention by attaching their name to an instruction or by making eye contact before giving instructions. (Be sensitive about eye contact as some pupils aren't comfortable with this)
- Provide a task planner – a visual reminder of the sequence of tasks or tick lists – so that the pupil can take responsibility for their tasks (see next page)

An example of a task planner

The task planner can be laminated so that the teacher or TA can write onto it what the pupil has to do. Instructions can be rubbed off and replaced with new ones in following lessons. Older pupils may be able to record at least the first instruction themselves. You can use 'traffic light' colours to provide additional visual clues about task sequence - the first in green, the next in orange, the last in red.

The task planner is a visual reminder but it also helps learners to feel more secure about the task at hand by breaking it down into manageable (and memorable) chunks.

Task Planner and Checklist
I need my:

Maths book ☐
Ruler ☐
Rubber ☐

First   Copy the title and date

Next   Do the sums 1 to 4

Then   Check the answers

Last   Write down homework tasks

Attention and concentration

Attention and concentration are two fundamental aspects of all learning in the classroom. Learners with dyspraxia have very poor attention and concentration skills. Although they do not have hearing difficulties, they may appear not to be listening and get distracted very easily. You may observe that they are very fidgety, moving constantly or rocking backward and forward. The main reasons for their attention and concentration difficulties are due to their inability to:

- Balance and fix their bodies to sit still for an extended period of time. They become fidgety as they are constantly trying to stabilise their bodies, which breaks their attention

- Filter out unwanted sounds and movements

- Process and follow the sequence of task instructions due to poor auditory sequential memory and processing difficulties. They may watch others for clues and lose attention and concentration

Strategies to improve attention and concentration

Attention difficulties can often look like 'naughtiness' and 'disruptiveness' on the part of the learner, so it is important to understand that pupils with dyspraxia have genuine difficulty with listening, attention and concentration. Even if you remind them about correct listening behaviour, they may still be unable to conform.

On the carpet, for instance, pupils may be moving, fidgeting, leaning on others and invading their classmates' personal space. Their behaviour will annoy their peers who want to listen, and it can disrupt the whole lesson. These pupils need different strategies to improve their attention and concentration.

- Be realistic and consistent about your approach and expectations. These learners are not able to listen or stay on tasks for an extended period of time
- Provide a quieter 'work area', away from auditory and visual distractions
- Provide short and structured tasks with legitimate short breaks or 'time out'
- Encourage learners to adopt the correct sitting position at their desks or on the carpet, with support for their backs
- Provide a 'fidget object' to help pupils to listen and concentrate better

Time management

Pupils with dyspraxia find it hard to understand the concept of time. Although they are able to read the time, they have significant difficulties in managing it effectively. It is difficult for them to judge how long tasks will take to complete or how much detail is required for a writing task. They may think they have worked for hours when they have, in fact, only worked for a short time. They may spend 20 minutes writing the date and title of a story and then run out of time to write anything else. Pupils who struggle with 'time sense' become more disorganised and stressed when they are under time pressure. They don't:

- Move from one task to another in a timely manner
- Understand the concepts of past and future events
- Maintain an adequate pace during writing tasks

Learners with dyspraxia may be perceived by others as 'slow' and 'lazy' but the problem is due to their poor internal sense of timing. They also feel frustrated because their written work does not reflect their true abilities; their lack of time awareness prevents them from being successful.

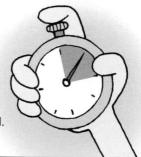

Developing a sense of time

Good time management skills are particularly important for secondary school pupils and are vital for exams. Poor timing and slow pacing have a negative impact on a learner's organisational and planning skills, as well as their ability to carry out everyday activities, such as moving from lesson to lesson, changing for PE, eating lunch etc. Through various 'timed' activities these learners can gradually develop a sense of time. Try the following:

- Provide more routine activities, as the familiarity of tasks will help to build confidence and provide opportunities for over-learning so that they can get quicker
- Use a clock in the classroom and refer to the time regularly for specific tasks
- Provide 'timed tasks' using a sand timer, buzzer or alarm clock
- Provide a visual timetable (use symbols or writing) or a task planner with times written on it, so that learners develop a sense of lesson length
- Encourage pupils to estimate how long a particular task will take to complete, then check with them how long it actually took to complete
- Be clear and explicit about the detail of tasks you expect within a set time

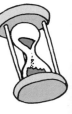

Build their time sense slowly and gradually, avoiding additional pressure.

Organisation

Good organisational skills are vital in all aspects of our lives, helping to develop independence in learning and daily living skills. Learners with dyspraxia have extreme difficulty in organising themselves, their belongings, their time and sequencing ideas and thoughts for writing. Although they try harder than their peers, they may struggle with basic organisational and self-help skills, which impacts negatively on their learning and confidence.

They often lose their personal belongings such as pens and pencils, forget to bring their PE kit or their homework, struggle to find the right books and equipment for lessons. They regularly miss deadlines, and their poor organisational skills make them feel anxious and embarrassed. They are often aware of their difficulties and hearing comments like *'clumsy'*, *'slow'* *'messy'* and *'always the last one'* from people around them is very frustrating and demoralising for them when they have this insight. Their organisational difficulties are due to:

- Immature and disorganised motor planning
- Poor motor memory
- Information processing difficulty
- Poor sense of timing

Self-organisation – the key to independence

Self-organisational skills are also linked with poor short-term memory and information overload. Routine, structure and an organised classroom reduce anxiety and help learners to feel secure and confident. Try to:

- Provide extra time for learners to plan, organise and complete their work
- Keep a pupil's belongings in a particular place
- Provide a written or visual timetable
- Provide a buddy system to support learners to organise tasks/equipment/homework and help them to navigate around secondary school
- Provide a checklist of equipment needed to start the task. For younger pupils, this could even be attached to the desk
- Liaise regularly with parents about homework/coursework, submission dates etc
- Discuss with parents how they might adapt their child's clothes and equipment appropriately, eg shoes with Velcro fastenings are easier to take on and off than ones with laces

Perceptual
Function

Seven senses!

Perception means the ability of the brain to make sense of the information it receives through different sensory organs. The brain constantly receives information from the environment through the senses and it then processes, interprets and organises it all in order to respond appropriately. Senses inform us whether something is dangerous or safe, near or far away, and allow us to engage and interact with our surroundings. Through sensory information and interactions we build our knowledge and understanding of our immediate environment and the world around us.

In addition to the five senses we all know, we have:

1. A **vestibular system** that contributes to our sense of balance
2. A **proprioceptive system** that keeps track of different parts of the body. It helps with body position awareness.

Pupils with dyspraxia have difficulty in receiving and *integrating* all the sensory information they receive and therefore struggle with a coherent response to sensory inputs. Their response may be slow and inaccurate and this can be the cause of learning and behaviour difficulties.

Sensory perception

Accurate perceptions and speedy responses are necessary to develop concepts and knowledge. Most pupils have already developed good perception skills by the time they start school but many pupils with dyspraxia have perception difficulties.

Not all aspects of sensory perception will be equally affected and each pupil will have a unique perception difficulty profile with specific weaknesses and strengths. You need to identify the nature of their perception difficulty in order to address their problem.

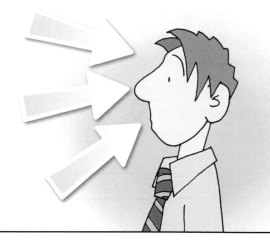

Making sense of it all

Sensory input we receive

Vision

Hearing

Touch

Smell

Balance

Proprioception

Taste

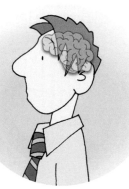

The **Brain** receives, processes, integrates information

We respond to information...

...with our actions in order to develop concepts and to gain knowledge, eg:

- Moving our eyes
- Co-ordinating our bodies
- Walking

Sensory integration

Every conscious movement we make relies on the interpretation of sensory input by the brain. Pupils with dyspraxia may have difficulty in receiving, interpreting, integrating, organising and processing their sensory inputs into actions: this is described as a **sensory integration difficulty**. Some pupils may have a delayed or dysfunctional sensory integration system.

Sensory integration problems occur when the brain:

• Does not receive accurate sensory inputs or sensory organs do not work together
• Is not able to process or relate the new information to any previous experiences, positive or negative
• Is slow in processing sensory information
• Has difficulty in organising and planning the sequence of actions
• Has difficulty in carrying out the right motor action

Visual perception

Visual perception is the ability of the brain to interpret and organise information that it receives through the eyes. It is not related to eyesight but to how one sees and makes sense of visual input. Some pupils with dyspraxia may have difficulty in receiving, interpreting and processing visual information into actions and this has an impact on their cognitive development. Their difficulty could be due to an inability to:

- Move both eyes in a co-ordinated way
- Receive correct and complete visual information
- Process visual information at speed
- Carry out eye tracking from left and right for reading and writing
- Co-ordinate the eyes and hands to perform simple motor actions, eg tying shoelaces

A difficulty in visual perception has a significant impact on learning as most of the learning in the classroom (about 85%) is visual.

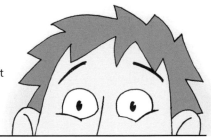

Aspects of visual perception

There are various aspects to visual perception. When they do not work efficiently in pupils with dyspraxia, it leads to a visual perception difficulty.

Visual discrimination – the ability to distinguish similarities and differences between shapes or objects

Visual memory and visual sequential memory – the ability to recall previous visual information

Visual spatial perception – the ability to understand the relationship of everything around us and the relationship between objects, eg 'next to', 'on'

Visuo-spatial memory – remembering the correct position of objects

Visual form constancy – the ability to recognise shapes or objects despite changes in size, colour and orientation

Visual figure ground – the ability to distinguish an object from its background

Visual closer – the ability to identify incomplete figures

Visual-motor integration – the ability to translate visual information into motor actions

Visual tracking – the ability to move the eyes in a controlled and sequential manner

Faulty visual perception and impact on learning

Accurate visual perception is vital to read, write and spell correctly and is necessary to carry out everyday living activities such as walking, dressing and eating.

Each learner with dyspraxia may have unique visual perceptual motor difficulties and they may have general problems in:

- Discriminating between different shapes, symbols, letters, words and numbers
- Interpreting pictures, diagrams, graphs or maps correctly
- Completing age-appropriate puzzles
- Matching letters, words and pictures
- Copying from the board or a worksheet
- Setting out maths problems correctly
- Reading accurately – they may miss lines or lose their place
- Discriminating prominent features in objects
- Attention to detail in a complicated and 'busy' picture

Visual perception management

You may need to refer a pupil with faulty visual perception to an ophthalmologist to identify the exact nature of their difficulty and to provide individualised interventions if you notice the child is showing signs of eye discomfort when they read. Be aware of their sitting position in the classroom and the glare from the sunlight as these can increase visual distortions and visual distress. Try to provide:

- Opportunities to practise visual search/scan using pictures, word searches
- Visually uncluttered worksheets
- Worksheets with large fonts and double spacing
- An angled board or a rigid A4 file for better visual attention
- Mechanical supports for reading eg reading ruler/window to help the pupil concentrate and focus on a few lines at a time instead of being overwhelmed by a whole block of text
- A variety of coloured overlays, which may help to reduce visual distress or visual contrasts – these are commercially available
- A multi-sensory approach to focus on visual aspects of letters/words
- A specific seating place, so that the pupil directly faces you and the board

Auditory perception

Children with dyspraxia may have good hearing but they may have problems
with various aspects of auditory perception, ie how the brain interprets what it hears.
Accurate auditory perception is vital for language and concept development and
phonological (letter sound) awareness, both of which are essential for developing
literacy skills. There are different aspects of auditory perception:

- **Auditory processing speed** – the ability to interpret and process what is heard at
  an appropriate speed
- **Auditory memory** – the ability to process and remember auditory information
- **Auditory sequential memory** – the ability to follow verbal
  instructions in a sequential order
- **Auditory discrimination** – the ability to distinguish
  similar sounds or words
- **Sequencing sounds** – hearing and recalling
  sequences of sounds, eg m-a-t
- **Sound localisation** – the ability to identify the
  source of a sound
- **Responsiveness to sound** – a learner may not
  respond appropriately to certain sounds (they
  may be over- or under-responsive)

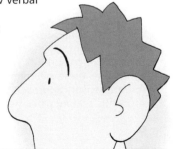

Faulty auditory perception and impact on learning

Pupils with auditory perception difficulties struggle to recognise subtle differences between sounds in words or speech and misinterpret the information they receive. Their problem is more obvious when they are in a noisy classroom environment and are listening to complex information. The pupil may be perceived as 'not listening' but due to their high level of auditory distractibility, they are unable to make sense of verbal information. They also struggle to establish links between new verbal information and previous knowledge. This affects their language and concept development. In class, you may observe they struggle to:

• Follow multiple-step instructions
• Listen and respond appropriately
• Interpret and process verbal information accurately with speed
• Develop spelling and comprehension skills

Auditory perception management

Learners with dyspraxia respond better when verbal information is supplemented with visual support. You may need to refer a pupil to an audiologist to identify the nature of their difficulty and to provide specific interventions. These are general classroom strategies you can try:

- Providing headphones to limit auditory distractions
- Teaching coping strategies so that they learn to ignore some background noises
- Giving step-by-step instructions using short and simple sentences with time in-between to process information
- Repeating the instructions slowly, without paraphrasing
- Making sensitive eye contact with the learner before giving instructions
- Providing brief written and verbal instructions to reduce auditory overload
- Making sure you have the pupil's attention before explaining key points
- Encouraging the learner to sit directly facing you
- Providing activities to improve language skills and vocabulary

Under-sensitive/hyposensitive

The touch, smell, balance and body awareness perceptions of some pupils with dyspraxia may be faulty and they may be over- or under-sensitive to sensory stimulation. Under- (hypo) sensitive learners may not receive adequate sensory feedback and so will seek extra sensory stimulation to function. They may:

- Act fidgety by fiddling or breaking equipment, chewing pencil/ pen tops, putting other objects in their mouths – all to get increased touch sensations
- Be messy in their eating habits, possibly due to a lack of touch sensation in their mouths
- Be slow in responding to verbal instructions, due to hyposensitivity of hearing
- Act impulsively, in order to seek out new sources of sensory stimulation

These learners need legitimate compensatory strategies to get extra sensory stimulation. Try providing them with a fiddle object to hold during listening sessions, a pen with a hard top or headphones to listen to music.

Over-sensitive/hypersensitive

Pupils who are over-sensitive to sensory stimuli can become over-excited by touch, sounds, smell, and light. They may be aggressive or disruptive, show impulsivity or hyperactivity and their motor performance may deteriorate further.

Such pupils may find it impossible to process information from more than one sense at a time and get distracted very easily. Some may 'switch off', look stubborn, get distressed or exhibit other behaviour problems. This is because they are unable to filter out unimportant sensory input and to prioritise the relevant one. They respond better in less sensory stimulating environments so you may observe that they are:

- Making noises, such as tapping with a pen or pencil, making humming noises to filter out other auditory distractions and to stay focused on task
- Covering their ears or exhibiting inappropriate behaviour when they are in a noisy environment
- Avoiding certain noisy areas or activities, eg PE/games, the dining hall at lunchtime, etc

Reducing sensory overload

Each pupil has different triggers for hypersensitivity, but with careful monitoring and observation, you may be able to identify these and act to reduce the frequency of inappropriate behaviour. You can reduce their sensory overload by providing:

- A quieter area to carry out tasks, away from visual and auditory sensory overload, eg with no visual distractions on the walls
- A clutter-free workstation and simple worksheets with reduced items
- Appropriate lighting in their work area – avoiding over-lit or under-lit environments
- Planned tasks that do not demand the use of more than one sense at a time, eg not requiring the student to listen at the same time as copying from the board
- A planned 'time out' session or a 'quiet corner' to calm the learner down when they are over excited or distressed

Touch perception

Touch perception or tactile perception is the ability to process information about the environment through the sense of touch. Through our skin, we feel environmental changes, eg temperature, pain, pressure etc and are able to discriminate those changes and learn those concepts. Pupils with dyspraxia may struggle to develop these concepts of feeling without added visual guidance.

Another aspect of touch perception is **touch discrimination** – the ability to distinguish different objects through touch. Young pupils begin to develop language concepts such as same/different, round/square, soft/hard, etc by using touch discrimination perception. Many older pupils touch and manipulate objects to understand the concepts of shapes and size in maths and the properties of materials in science, for example.

Pupils with dyspraxia who have a poor sense of touch cannot discriminate objects through touching alone; they need additional sensory information, such as visual guidance. They may also be hypersensitive or hyposensitive to touch. Accurate touch feedback is necessary to develop concepts and to understand our environment and the world.

Over- or under-sensitivity to touch

Under-sensitivity to touch
Children who are under-sensitive to touch and pain may injure themselves without realising and have higher pain threshold levels. Their physical play may be quite hurtful for others as they do not get the same pressure feedback as their peers. They may have poor awareness of the position of their limbs without being guided by vision. They constantly seek physical contact by touching others, putting things in their mouth, etc. Giving them a fiddling object, squeezy ball or a pen with a hard top to chew can provide the touch sensation they need.

Over-sensitivity to touch
Learners with a high level of tactile sensitivity to people, texture, food, temperature may overreact to physical contact with their peers. They do not like to be touched or hugged and find it very threatening when others are in close proximity. They do not like to line up in queues, play team sports and may not like the feeling of certain textures, such as sand, play dough, clothes labels. Be aware of the materials they are over-sensitive to and encourage them to sit at the end of the carpet or to line up at the end to minimise physical contact.

Distance, depth and lateralisation

Some learners with dyspraxia may have faulty perceptions of distance, depth and lateralisation, which will have an impact on their cognitive functioning and learning.

Distance perception – the ability to perceive the distance between yourself and other objects. Pupils may over- or under-estimate distance, which can cause problems in crossing roads as they misjudge the distance between the cars and oncoming traffic. They need to be encouraged to use more of their auditory and visual perceptions to compensate for their difficulties, eg hearing and looking for oncoming traffic, or crossing only at safe crossings.

Depth perception – the ability to perceive the world in three dimensions. Pupils may struggle to use PE apparatus and to perform everyday tasks – like climbing stairs – that require this skill. They may endanger themselves if they are not adequately supervised and can benefit from teaching on safety awareness using visual aids.

Distance, depth and lateralisation

Lateralisation

In the majority of right-handed people, the left side of the brain is responsible for controlling the right side of the body and the right side of the brain is responsible for left side of the body. Some pupils with dyspraxia do not have established hand dominance and, because of a lack of co-ordination between the two sides of their body, they struggle with 'bilateral integration' tasks. These include writing and using a knife and fork.

It is more difficult to improve bilateral integration the older a pupil gets but using these 'midline crossing' activities with younger pupils will help to improve their bilateral integration:

- Ball activities – catching and throwing ball using both hands, bouncing a ball using both hands. Provide variable ball sizes and distance to match the pupil's ability
- Beading/threading activities – picking and holding the beads in one hand and using the other hand to thread
- Cutting with scissors – holding and turning paper with one hand and using scissors in the other hand to cut
- Picking up objects with the right hand from the left side and moving an object to their right side, repeating with the left hand and an object on the right side

Smell and taste, orientation

Smell and taste
Many pupils with dyspraxia have a heightened sense of taste and smell; as a result they may dislike the smell of certain foods. They may also dislike the texture of certain foods in their mouth. For instance, they may not like solid and liquid foods mixed together and may avoid eating them at the same time. It is important that the school is fully aware of any food sensitivities and liaises regularly with parents to ensure children do not react inappropriately to certain foods. Other children may be unable to distinguish between edible and non-edible objects and put everything in their mouths. You may need to seek further advice from the school health adviser about a pupil's eating habits.

Orientation
Some pupils may have problems distinguishing left from right. They may have difficulty in following directional commands in PE and may need physical guidance to learn directional movements. Try to teach one direction at a time and make sure this is fully established before you teach the next direction.

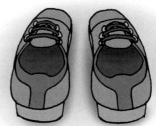

Vestibular or balance system

The vestibular (balance) system enables us to maintain our balance and posture and to cope with unexpected movements without falling. The balance-controlling senses are located in the inner ear and help us to maintain an upright position against gravity. Postural stability and balance are important in gross motor activities such as running, jumping, stopping and changing directions with confidence. Good postural balance is also needed to carry out fine motor activities, such as writing. As pupils get older, the balance system becomes more refined. Learners with dyspraxia have an under-developed balance system and you may observe:

- Poor co-ordination
- An inability to maintain an upright position
- Slumping over a desk or supporting the head with their hands
- Clumsiness, tripping over or bumping into things
- Uncontrolled running, jumping and spinning actions
- Excessive head movements, hand-flapping
- Difficulties walking on uneven ground

Activities focusing on developing balance and co-ordination can be found on page 84.

Spatial awareness

Spatial perception is awareness of our body position in relation to other objects and the surrounding environment. By exploring the space around them, infants start to gain a sense of their own position and an understanding of the relationship between objects as well as distance, direction, and language concepts such as up/down under/over and big/small.

Learners with dyspraxia often have poor spatial awareness as they do not receive the correct sensory feedback from their muscles and nerves. They may have difficulty in adjusting their bodies when they encounter objects in the space around them. This leads to lots of accidents, such as bumping into people or objects, or tripping over, which can, in turn, cause feelings of failure and low self-esteem. Learners may have difficulty staying within their personal space and there could be increased danger in practical lessons, eg science, PE. Try to:

- Provide as much space as possible around the learner at their desks or, with younger children, on the carpet to avoid them bumping into others
- Provide a visual boundary on the carpet to delineate a learner's own space

Secondary
Consequences

Psychological difficulties

In addition to the direct areas of difficulties described in previous chapters, some pupils with dyspraxia develop psychological, social and emotional difficulties, which can have a long-term impact on their lives. These are known as 'secondary consequences'.

Pupils may struggle with social interactions, have difficulty making friends and coping with everyday life. They risk becoming socially isolated and depressed. Some pupils become victims of bullying or start to develop behaviour difficulties.

Pupils with dyspraxia need support not only to cope with the academic demands of the classroom but to develop their non-academic skills, such as social and friendship skills. Focus on developing their emotional wellbeing, so that they feel confident and their self-esteem improves.

The failure cycle

Failures in the classroom and feedback they receive from peers and significant others can lead some pupils with dyspraxia to develop negative perceptions about themselves. They harbour feelings of incompetence, inadequacy and unhappiness; they become withdrawn and lonely, with poor self-esteem and confidence.

Examples of emotional and behavioural difficulties include:

- Feeling inadequate/worthless
- Low self-esteem
- Severe depression
- Mood swings
- Bedwetting

- Refusal to attend school
- Anxiety, stress
- Anger and frustration
- Lack of interest and motivation
- Social isolation

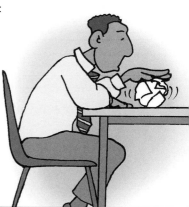

Behaviour difficulties

Jamal, a Year 9 pupil, is always in trouble with his teachers. His English teacher describes him as very fidgety and he is often disruptive in lessons. His behaviour includes constantly moving in his seat, shouting out other pupils' names, making inappropriate noises in lessons. Jamal is extremely disorganised and forgets to bring the right books to his lessons. He finds it hard to listen during whole class discussions and loses concentration. Although his handwriting is good, he struggles to start written tasks as he finds it difficult to sequence ideas – he gets easily frustrated and then 'lashes out' in the classroom. Other teachers have remarked that in their lessons he appears to lack motivation and interest and gives up easily.

Unmotivated	Disruptive
Anxious	Behaving as a class clown
Frustrated	Not listening
Stressed	Making silly noises

Jamal is showing many typical examples of inappropriate behaviour exhibited by some pupils with dyspraxia. There are often genuine reasons for their behavioural difficulties, which are explored in the following pages.

Behaviour difficulties – why?

It is easy to misunderstand the pupil with dyspraxia, perceiving inappropriate classroom behaviour as naughtiness. In reality, there may be a number of underlying reasons for their behaviour:

- Difficulty in processing incoming information, organising ideas/thoughts and maintaining time and pace for written tasks

- Sensory sensitivity – senses are over/under stimulated during lessons, making it difficult to listen

- Inability to work co-operatively with others due to a lack of social understanding

- Some pupils have overlapping difficulties with ADHD, which cause a lack of attention and concentration as well as impulsivity. They may fidget due to an inability to control their balance and posture and sitting still may be extremely difficult for them

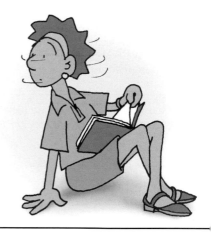

Strategies for behaviour improvement

As we have seen, fidgeting, emotional and behavioural difficulties may not always be the pupil's fault.

It is important to observe and analyse the pupil's behaviour in various contexts, both inside and outside the classroom. With older pupils, it is helpful to discuss the issues sensitively and in private, away from their peers. Talk to them about their feelings and emotions and try to help them to understand why they are behaving in that way. Have realistic expectations of their behaviour and offer options and choices that are appropriate to their level of skill and understanding.

By analysing and adjusting the task and environment carefully it may be possible to manage the inappropriate behaviour. For example, it may be possible to reduce the length of listening sessions or break down the tasks into smaller chunks by providing visual cues of tasks.

Praise pupils for their efforts – this will develop their motivation and confidence. Try to take a constructive rather than a punitive approach to their behavioural difficulties.

Difficulty with social interactions

Emily is a Year 8 pupil. She is overweight and very uncoordinated with her movements. She does not have many friends. Her teachers have noticed that she appears isolated and lonely during break times and does not join in with playground games. Emily appears withdrawn and has told her teachers that she prefers to avoid interacting with her peers because they call her names. On occasion, she feels so unhappy and anxious that she tells her mother she is feeling too unwell to come to school.

This is sadly an all too common story amongst pupils with dyspraxia. They have significant difficulty in interacting with others during unstructured social situations due to:

- An inability to understand and follow unwritten non-verbal complex social cues/rules and expectations
- An inability to rectify social mistakes
- Poor performance in motor-based team activities, such as games/sports
- Difficulties with subtle language and communication skills. Where pupils have a very literal understanding they cannot respond appropriately to idioms and playground jokes

Signs of social interaction difficulty

Jason's Maths teacher describes him as a 'day dreamer', who likes to be on his own and does not participate in group discussions. During group work, Jason copies the silly behaviour of other pupils, eg name calling, making noises with his ruler, verbal exchanges during listening time.

Most of the inappropriate behaviours exhibited by pupils with dyspraxia, like Jason, are due to a lack of social understanding. Pupils are easily led by others and situations can sometimes get out of hand. There are many signs of social interaction difficulty, some of which are outlined below:

- Withdrawn, lonely, unhappy and disruptive
- Interrupts conversation and is perceived as 'odd 'or 'rude' by others
- Shows rigidity in social contexts, such as in games
- Unable to cope with winning/losing games, exhibits excessive emotions
- Follows certain rituals or other obsessive behaviour
- Plays with younger pupils rather than their peers

It is important to identify the pupil's specific difficulties by observing them in different situations in order to target how best to teach them the social skills they need.

Developing positive social interactions

Social skills are complex and multi-faceted and pupils with dyspraxia cannot learn the unwritten social rules simply by observing others. They need to be taught how to communicate, how to relate to others more effectively and how to read and respond to non-verbal communication. They need opportunities to learn and practise these skills in a safe environment.

Try to identify the individual aspects of social behaviour they need to improve. Provide positive social experiences through structured activities, such as computer clubs and other lunchtime/after-school clubs, facilitated by an adult, where they can share common interests with their peers.

In some cases, a 'mentoring' system could be used to support social skills development. Use specific games/activities, which focus on developing appropriate social skills, such as how to understand and respond to body language and emotions.

Encourage pupils to join activities they enjoy for positive social interactions and fun, which is important for their wellbeing.

Developing and maintaining friendships

Sunil told me he did not have any friends, even though he had been at the same school since Reception and was now in Year 6. He even struggled to tell me the names of the pupils who sat next to him. He was telling jokes which others did not find funny and they thought of him as 'odd' and 'silly'.

The social gap between pupils with dyspraxia and their peers widens as they get older. They struggle to relate to their peers and to develop and maintain friendships over time. Their inadequate and immature social skills, uncoordinated movements and clumsiness all have a negative impact on potential friendships. What makes things worse is that they often do not know how to rectify the situation, eg by apologising when they bump into others or knock over equipment.

- Provide planned opportunities for developing friendships, such as grouping pupils together who have similar interests or hobbies
- Provide 'Circle of Friends' material to help develop and maintain friendships between pupils (see page 123 for further information)

Bullying

Pupils with motor co-ordination difficulties are often bullied in school because of their slowness and clumsiness; they can become very unpopular. Bullying can start at any age and can be verbal, emotional or physical. It has a profound effect on a pupil's learning, social, psychological and emotional development. One study found that 75% of children who were bullied had co-ordination problems. A wide range of anti-bullying strategies can be found in the *Stop Bullying Pocketbook* written by Kidscape founder Michele Elliott. In addition:

- 'Circle Time' or role play sessions can be sensitively used with the whole class to discuss issues and the impact of bullying to develop understanding and empathy from peers
- Provide supervision during unstructured times, eg lunch and break times
- Develop and discuss the school's ethos of valuing and respecting everybody and reinforce the school's anti-bullying policy
- Provide a support network, 'playground pal' scheme, or mentoring system
- Develop staff awareness of bullying, and address problems that arise as soon as possible

Self-esteem and emotional success

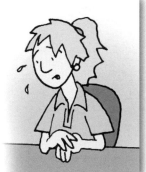

Lucy, a Year 5 pupil, was diagnosed with dyspraxia about 2 years ago. She is very keen to please adults and wants to be liked by her peers. Her understanding is very limited and she is able to produce very little written work. Lucy shows eagerness to contribute during whole class discussions. However, her responses are often totally unrelated to what is being asked. Even with differentiated questions, Lucy struggles to respond correctly. Sometimes, her responses initiate laughter amongst her peers. During my observations, Lucy approached me for help and told me that she was 'thick' because she could not work and explain things like others.

Like Lucy, most learners with dyspraxia are aware of their difficulties and are aware of being perceived negatively by others. Try to use their strengths to instil an '*I am good at ....*', approach, so that they see themselves positively and share their interests, hobbies and achievements with their peers, so that *they* can see them positively too. This will improve their self-esteem, social interactions, confidence and learning.

Problems with Motor Memory

Movement and motor planning

Performing any movement requires effective sensory perception, motor planning and motor co-ordination. Every day, we perform numerous complex living activities automatically and without thinking – walking, tying shoelaces, writing, driving, etc. This is dependent on a part of the brain, known as the **motor** or **muscle memory**, that stores information about how to do these tasks. The more we repeat an action, the better it is stored in our motor memory until eventually we do not have to think about it anymore. For example, it would not be difficult for you to write your name with your eyes closed because the information about that movement is stored in your motor memory and does not require visual guidance.

Pupils with dyspraxia have poor motor memory. They have difficulty storing their previous motor actions and so are required to make conscious planning decisions about movements. They need visual guidance to perform even simple daily tasks, such as brushing their teeth or doing up buttons. As a result, their movements, rather than fluent and automatic, tend to be slow and awkward, lacking adaptability and flexibility.

Sequencing and movement speed

All movement tasks are the result of a sequence of actions performed in the correct order to reach a goal. Just as our motor memory can store the actions we perform, it can also store information about the correct *sequence* of movements needed to fulfil a purposeful goal.

Activities that require a number of sequential actions, such as getting dressed, can be particularly difficult for pupils with dyspraxia. Their motor performances become slow, hesitant and disorganised, and they may end up putting on their shoes before their trousers, for example.

With opportunities for repetition of tasks, children with dyspraxia are more likely to be able to develop speed and fluency with their sequencing.

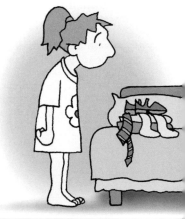

Difficulty with generalisation and multi-tasking

As the subconscious motor memory gets more adept at facilitating fast, fluent and automatic actions in the right sequence, it also allows multi-tasking. You are only able to do more than one thing at a time if you can perform individual actions without conscious thought, for instance tying your laces whilst talking to someone else.

Even after performing a particular motor task several times, pupils with dyspraxia may struggle to generalise learned tasks in different contexts. They have significant difficulty in multi-tasking, such as listening whilst taking notes, because they still need to think about and plan learned tasks in a new context. As a result, their tasks become laboured and slow in both reaction and response time and their performance does not reach an automatic level.

Gross motor skills

We regularly perform a range of 'big' motor actions – walking, swimming, running, cycling. These are called **gross motor movements**, as distinct from 'small' motor actions, like writing and cutting, which are known as **fine motor movements** (see page 88). Some pupils with dyspraxia have both gross and fine motor difficulties; others have *either* gross *or* fine motor difficulties.

When the large muscles which are required to carry out gross motor activities do not work in a co-ordinated way, movements look immature and clumsy. (Eg, an awkward gait when running.) Pupils with gross motor difficulty may lack stamina and have poor exercise tolerance. The main reasons for gross motor difficulties are:

- Postural instability, balance and co-ordination
- Poor body awareness and lack of integration between left and right sides of the body
- Sensory processing/integrating and motor planning difficulties
- Poor organisational skills

It is important to identify the nature of a pupil's gross motor difficulties through observations. Some pupils will require further assessment from a physiotherapist for a specialist individualised intervention programme.

Physical education and games

Taking part in PE, games and dance lessons is one of the most challenging activities for pupils with gross motor difficulties. They soon become aware of their limitations and tend to avoid such activities for fear of failure, leading to social isolation and loneliness. They become less physically fit, yet they need opportunities to develop their gross motor and co-ordination skills and confidence.

It has been established through various studies that physical activity can have a substantial impact on the broader development of pupils with specific learning difficulties like dyspraxia. It enables pupils to improve their physical fitness, co-ordination, balance, spatial awareness, social and friendship skills and also cognitive processing skills, such as attention, concentration and organisation.

As pupils cannot easily learn or develop skills from watching others, they need access to a differentiated PE curriculum, flexible teaching and learning strategies, organisational support, and encouragement to improve their skills, confidence and participation.

Difficulties with physical education and games

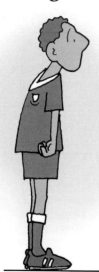

I was asked to observe a Year 3 boy, Sam, in his PE lesson. I arrived shortly before the start of the lesson when the class was getting changed. Sam followed others to get his PE kit from the cloakroom but then struggled to find his kit hanging on his peg. He had trouble undoing the buttons of his shirt and unzipping his trousers. He was painfully slow and found it extremely difficult to get changed for PE independently. He was watching others and got distracted by them but his peers had no problem getting changed whilst talking. When his teacher said 'Come on Sam, hurry up! Everybody is waiting for you', Sam felt more pressurised. He was the last to join the line. Visibly exhausted, his PE shirt was on back-to-front with his right and left shoes mixed up. His peers were laughing at him but Sam looked totally confused, not realising what he had done wrong. Sam struggled to participate throughout the lesson. He couldn't understand instructions and was last to be chosen when the class was asked to work in pairs or groups.

What support can you offer?

We have all met pupils like Sam, who need support to develop their time sense, self-help, organisational and gross motor skills to increase their participation in PE and games.

Pupils like Sam need encouragement to take part in non-competitive games/sports. Swimming, cycling, and walking will all improve their gross motor skills and their level of physical activity and stamina. You can develop time awareness by providing timed activities where they compete against themselves. Also, try to offer:

- A differentiated PE curriculum, such as walking along a straight line, hopping, jumping, cycling, standing on one leg, etc
- An achievable, small-step, individualised development programme targeting specific skills

To support organisational skills during PE and games, build in extra time before and after PE lessons to get changed, and liaise with parents about labelled, easy-to-take-off-and-put-on clothes, such as elasticated trousers and Velcro-fastened shoes.

Movement and cognitive development

There is a strong correlation between the physical attributes of balance and co-ordination and a pupil's ability to read, write, spell and copy, because learning these skills requires both cognitive ability and efficient motor performance. Movement is known to enhance both physical and cognitive development; in other words:

> **The development of motor skills is crucial to the development of cognitive skills.**

In addition to the classroom strategies discussed in previous chapters, try to provide some daily motivating and enjoyable movement activities, which can be fun for pupils with dyspraxia and will help to improve their motor-based learning and develop language concepts such as under/over, left/right. Regular scheduled movement activities can also help the pupil to re-focus and continue work to completion.

It is important that you appreciate their efforts and praise them accordingly; not necessarily measuring them against outcomes that they are not always able to achieve.

Improving balance and co-ordination

Balance is the one of the most important senses relating to movement and some pupils with dyspraxia have poor balance. When they carry out any movement activities, they struggle to maintain or regain balance quickly and fall over very easily. They find it difficult to sit up straight. Try to provide these gross motor activities to improve balance and coordination:

- Crawling, climbing, hopping, jumping, obstacle courses
- Walking on a balance beam, wide to narrow
- Standing on one foot with eyes open and eyes closed
- Heel-toe walking, moving between objects
- Jumping with feet together, jumping sideways, star jumping, jumping into hoops
- Standing on one foot, walking on uneven ground
- Running with change of speed and direction
- Catching and throwing a ball while jumping

Improved balance and co-ordination leads to increased confidence and academic achievement. Note that some pupils with significant difficulty may require specialist physiotherapy to develop their balance and co-ordination.

Improving balance and co-ordination

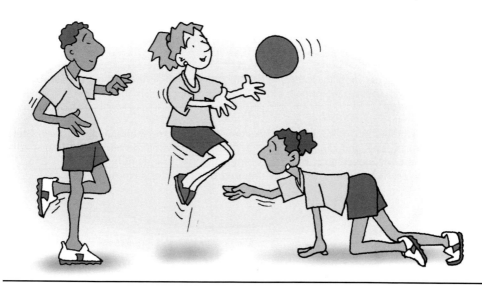

Hyper-mobility and low muscle tone (hypotonia)

Some people with dyspraxia have hyper-mobile joints; others may have hypotonia or low muscle tone.

Pupils with hyper-mobility syndrome will 'fix' parts of their limbs to increase stability. They may also have pain in their joints. They often write in small print but will have good control.

Pupils with low muscle tone have difficulties sitting up and maintaining posture. They may look 'floppy' and can struggle to keep their bodies still, perhaps exhibiting excessive body movements. You might notice this particularly during assembly and listening sessions where children are required to sit still for a length of time.

With thanks to Dr. Amanda Kirby for advice and guidance on these conditions.

Hand dominance and left-handers

A clear hand preference for many children with dyspraxia may not be fully established until quite late; they may swap hands to carry out different tasks. Pupils with dyspraxia who use their left hands may encounter difficulties when seated next to right-hand dominant pupils. Check their seating position in class and provide adequate space around them when they carry out group work. You can also train left-handed pupils to think by themselves about their seating area to prevent elbow-clashing in the classroom.

Remember that pupils who use their left hands may have difficulty in copying demonstrated movements from right-handed teachers or peers. Provide physical guidance using their body/hands to carry out the correct movements.

Fine motor skills

Fine motor skills refer to small muscle movements which work together in an organised way to carry out small and delicate tasks. These include writing, drawing, cutting, painting and manipulating objects, which all require finger manipulation, strength, control, dexterity and co-ordination.

As some pupils with dyspraxia do not have adequate finger strength, grip and pinch, they struggle with fine motor tasks. The physical activities below will help develop their fine motor skills and the mechanical aspects of writing:

- **Finger strength development exercises** – bursting bubbles in bubble wrap, squeezing and releasing rubber balls of increasing tension, pop-apart beads, paper tearing and crumpling
- **Finger manipulation** – threading beads, pegboard patterns, using paperclips, jigsaw puzzles, clay modelling, tracing, finger painting
- **Finger control** – touching each fingertip to the thumb in sequence
- **Fine motor co-ordination** – cutting, tying shoelaces, Lego, jigsaws

Developing fine motor skills

Difficulties with fine motor skills are very common in pupils with dyspraxia and they can be directly impacted by problems with gross motor skills. For example, handwriting – a fine motor skill – requires good balance, posture and co-ordination, which are all gross motor skills. Learners with dyspraxia usually have poor balance, co-ordination and posture, all of which affect the legibility of their writing.

In addition, pupils with dyspraxia tend to have difficulties with grapho-motor skills – these are a combination of cognitive, perceptual and fine motor skills which enable pupils to write. To develop grapho-motor skills, pupils need access to hand exercises, handwriting practice and letter-formation programmes.

Remember that these pupils need a more concentrated effort than their peers to carry out fine motor tasks and as a result they tire easily.

Problems with handwriting

Children who struggle with the mechanics of handwriting find it difficult to demonstrate their knowledge and skills.

You may observe that pupils with dyspraxia perform better during handwriting practice sessions compared to free-writing tasks that involve thinking, sequencing and recording. When they are not concentrating exclusively on their handwriting, it often reverts to being messy and illegible, with erratic letter sizing, formation and spacing. This could be due to a difficulty in multi-tasking as well as to fundamental problems with motor skills and a poor motor memory affecting writing automaticity.

In addition, the handwriting of children with motor difficulties often deteriorates rapidly during long handwriting tasks due to fatigue from over-tight pen/pencil grip or pressing too hard on the paper. Poor technique may make their wrist ache and their writing hand become hot and sweaty. Although pupils with dyspraxia may concentrate harder than their peers to complete written tasks, their writing often does not reflect their cognitive ability.

Motor aspects of handwriting

Neat handwriting and a reasonable writing pace are significant challenges for pupils with dyspraxia. Although they often have average or above average cognitive ability, their perceptual and motor difficulties have an enormous impact on the presentation, fluency and speed of their handwriting. Their handwriting difficulty is due to a combination of factors:

- **Poor motor control** – an inability to make the correct fine muscle movements for handwriting
- **Poor 'body sense'** – an inability to keep track of where their fingers are when writing
- **Poor motor memory** – difficulty in remembering how to move the finger muscles
- **Poor postural control** – difficulty with central stability
- **Perceptual difficulty** – difficulty in leaving spaces between words

Developing writing skills

For pupils with dyspraxia who are required to complete long writing tasks, the following strategies can improve their engagement:

- Breaking down long written tasks into smaller chunks to make them more achievable. Depending on the pace of learner, each chunk can be completed at different times
- Making sure the paper or book is positioned correctly, preferably to their writing side. Clipboards and bulldog clips can be used to temporarily secure the paper during the writing task
- Providing an angled board or an angled folder for better positioning
- Providing appropriate writing equipment, eg thick pencil, appropriate pencil grips, writing spacer
- Placing dots at the left hand side of each new line to indicate the beginning of each line and to support directionality
- Encouraging the correct sitting position and finger warming-up exercises before writing tasks

Writing and alternative methods to record work

Even with improved access to technology, a large proportion of the school day involves writing and note-taking by hand. It is therefore important to offer opportunities to better reflect the abilities of pupils with dyspraxia and maintain their motivation. Have realistic expectations of written tasks and focus on the *quality* of the content rather than the quantity or format of presentation. Similarly, when assessing written work, focus on one aspect of their writing at a time, eg accuracy of content, not spelling, handwriting, presentation and grammar all at once.

Try to keep written recording to a minimum or reduce the need for recording by hand by:

- Providing cloze sentences, comic strips, speech bubbles, diagrams, labelling, graphs, tables and charts, drama/role play, posters or leaflets
- Encouraging pupils to use 'Mind maps', 'Concept maps' or other forms of visual representation (eg sequencing pictures/sentences) to retell stories or events
- Encouraging learners to use alternative forms of recording, eg a word processors with read-aloud software, dictaphones, tape recorders or scribes

Sequencing ideas and thoughts

In writing, the correct sequencing of ideas and thoughts is essential. To be able to write ideas and thoughts on paper, pupils need to have efficient cognitive, perceptual and motor abilities. Some pupils with dyspraxia are very good verbally but have trouble recording their ideas and thoughts on paper in a sequential way. Their difficulties are due to:

- Poor organisational and sequencing skills
- Poor language concepts
- Poor short-term memory, reading and comprehension skills
- Word-finding difficulties – inability to recall words from their long-term memory
- Poor semantic knowledge

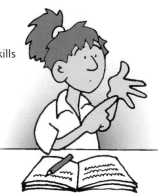

Mind maps and concept maps can help them to link their thoughts and sequence their ideas; sequence cards/activities can teach them the sequence of a story and writing frames or story frames can demonstrate ways to structure their writing

Learning New Skills

Learning styles

Children develop their language and thinking skills, physical co-ordination, social skills and self-confidence through movement by looking (visual), listening (auditory) and doing (kinaesthetic). These are the three main learning styles. Kinaesthetic learners are also known as motor learners.

Most pupils have one or two learning styles and can adapt these depending on the task at hand. For pupils with dyspraxia, learning new tasks is problematic as they are less flexible and can only learn when material is presented to them in their preferred learning style.

It is important to identify their preferred learning styles and increase their awareness of how to use these more effectively in their learning. They will usually need visual and physical guidance on how to complete tasks.

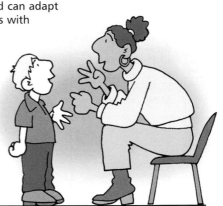

Teaching and learning techniques

As well as identifying the preferred learning style of pupils with dyspraxia and using a multi-sensory approach, you can implement a number of other practical strategies that will aid their learning:

- Provide direct teaching for specific skills
- Create opportunities for 'hands on' work
- Teach them visualisation and verbalisation techniques
- Encourage them to look for links between objects, position, shape and associations, such as the 'Mind map' technique
- Encourage them to use rhyme or association of words to aid recall
- Teach them how to link new information with previous knowledge and make sure that the new learning is built securely on what they already know and can do
- Teach specific memory techniques, eg 'chunking' information
- Provide opportunities to practise learned skills, so they feel a sense of achievement

Assessing functional skills

As teachers we are expected to carry out our own assessments and take action to address a pupil's learning needs. It is, therefore, crucial that we have a good understanding and awareness of the characteristics of dyspraxia for early identification and for timely intervention.

Form an holistic view of a pupil's difficulties by taking into account the types of problems the child encounters, as well as the interactions they experience, both at school and at home. You can then look at the 'big picture' and assess how dyspraxia interferes with development in the areas of:

- Organisation
- Social skills and play
- Physical and motor development
- Language and communication

- Cognition
- Emotion
- Perception
- Self-help and independence

Further assessment

If you suspect you have a pupil in your class with dyspraxia, it is important to have a discussion with the pupil's parents so that their child can be referred for a medical assessment. As dyspraxia is a medical diagnosis, the pupil will need a number of investigations to:

- Ensure the correct primary diagnosis is made
- Identify any overlapping learning difficulties
- Identify any other medical conditions such as cerebral palsy, as the interventions or strategies for conditions like this are different for pupils with dyspraxia alone
- Check hearing and vision – a referral can then be made to the Sensory Impairments Service if necessary
- Facilitate referrals to other services (see next page)

The multi-disciplinary team will identify each learner's unique set of difficulties. Some may need more individualised specialist interventions than others.

Specialist interventions

The previous chapters have outlined general strategies to support pupils with their motor development and language skills, whilst recognising that some pupils need more specialist input. Following the initial medical assessment of a pupil, a referral may be made by the school's SEN co-ordinator to any of the following services:

- **Physiotherapy** – to focus on developing the pupil's gross motor skills, balance, strength, posture stability and hand-eye co-ordination
- **Occupational therapy** – to focus on developing a pupil's fine motor co-ordination and grapho-motor control. Occupational therapists also provide sensory integration therapy, which is geared towards primary school children to improve perceptual skills, which are necessary for their learning
- **Speech and language therapy** – to provide support with developing speech sounds or to provide advice to develop the pupil's receptive language skills

Any of the specialist interventions provided may cross over, depending on the therapist's skills and training and the individual needs of the pupil. Interventions may be delivered in specialist clinics as well as provided for in the school and home environments.

Difficulties with reading, spelling and maths

We have seen how you can support learners to develop their attention/concentration, organisation and motivation – these are prerequisites for developing more complex reading and writing, spelling and maths skills.

Reading

Some students with dyspraxia are good at reading; others struggle to read accurately and fluently and may be perceived as 'reluctant readers'. They may be slow or hesitant, lose attention and concentration or rub their eyes a lot while reading. They may miss individual words or whole lines, or may be unable to read words in isolation whilst being able to read them in context. To facilitate reading accuracy and fluency, try to:

- Teach vocabulary separately – the subject vocabulary can be written on different colour cards for easy retrieval and learning
- Provide enlarged reading text on pastel coloured paper to reduce visual stress
- Provide a sloping reading surface and opportunities for 'pair reading'
- Use appropriate reading software to increase motivation to read, eg Clicker 5 (see page 124)

Activities to improve the mechanics of reading

Whether learners with dyspraxia struggle with the mechanics of reading or with comprehension, both are due to poor short-term memory and processing difficulties. Poor reading fluency can be due to poor visual discrimination (inability to discriminate similar shapes of letter/words), problems with eye tracking (both eyes do not follow a line of print smoothly), sequencing or directional problems (inability to read consistently from left to right). The following exercises and activities will help to improve decoding and copying skills:

- Visual tracking/eye movement activities (for tracking moving objects horizontally and vertically) – rolling a ball left to right, computer games
- Directional awareness activities – following a moving finger from left to right or reading from a computer screen with a cursor moving left to right across the screen
- Hand-eye co-ordination exercises – throwing and catching balls/beanbags, puzzles, picking up and posting coins into a slot
- Visual discrimination activities – snap games, spot the difference, dominos

Spelling

Pupils with dyspraxia often struggle with spelling due to difficulties with visual perception or with visual and motor memory and sequencing.

Their problems include:
* Reading/remembering shapes, sequencing letters
* Substitution of words that are formed with similar motor movements (for example, r/b/h or d/g/a), when they write or spell
* Inability to articulate sounds and organise them into words (due to poor muscle co-ordination of their mouth), which is reflected in their spelling
* Difficulties reading their own writing for a visual check of their spelling

You can develop spelling confidence and competence by:
* Using activities to improve visual discrimination and visual sequencing memory, eg pattern copying, threading coloured beads, word search activities
* Teaching them the visual aspects of words, eg their *shape*
* Providing spell checkers and word lists for their independent writing
* Using a multi-sensory approach to teach spelling

Maths

Most pupils with dyspraxia have the expected conceptual understanding of mathematics for their age, but they struggle to apply this understanding and record it manually. Their difficulties are mainly due to poor visual perceptual skills, lack of spatial awareness and sequential memory problems.

Pupils find it difficult to recall number patterns and record their written work in the correct order. They struggle to set out maths calculations correctly, which affects their answers. They are unable to recognise the value of each number by its position and cannot carry numbers across the columns in their correct position.

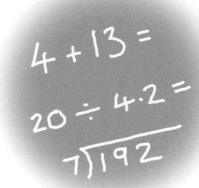

Maths Strategies

- Teach **spatial and directional skills** by using directional games in PE and pegboard games to teach horizontal, vertical and diagonal directions and spacing

- Teach **maths concepts** using various games and activities, such as hanging socks on a washing line in pairs or 'odd one out' to demonstrate odd and even, and cutting activities to convey the concepts of whole and halves

- Teach **maths operations** such as addition/subtraction using visual aids

- Teach **calculation strategies** using highlighter pens on columns of hundreds, tens and units to show where to begin calculations

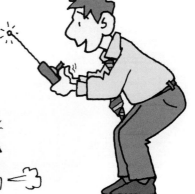

Study skills

Pupils with dyspraxia need additional support to develop their study skills*.
They may find it difficult to organise their time, take notes and understand and retain
information.

You can teach them various study techniques, eg mind mapping, concept mapping,
flow charts and higher order reading techniques to extract information. Try to:

- Provide them with a 'study buddy'/ 'learning buddy'
- Provide lists of key vocabulary/ subject vocabulary
- Provide them with their own copy of each text
- Encourage them to use highlighter pens to mark key points
- Provide enlarged diagrams/ worksheets with diagrams, which are easier to label
- Provide extra time for writing and drawing
- Encourage them to use a tape recorder or teach them how to take notes

Study skills and learning techniques are covered in more detail in the **Learning to Learn and
Accelerated Learning Pocketbooks*

How to develop study skills

Efficient study skills are essential for academic success. Exam times are very stressful for all learners; even more so for learners with dyspraxia. More guidance and support may be required to maintain motivation and to boost revision techniques, note-taking and exam strategies.

All dyspraxic learners will benefit from:

- A study timetable with times written on it
- Routine, structure and support with their organisational skills
- An area where they can study that is quiet and free of distractions
- Structured short study sessions with regular breaks
- Acquiring the habit of reading through study material several times and repeating it back
- Highlighting different aspects/key points with different coloured pens
- Making notes on important information/ facts and linking these using mind-mapping techniques, visualisation, word association and mnemonics
- Studying with peers and reviewing together what they have learned or read
- Recording information using a variety of media

ICT skills

Encourage learners with dyspraxia to develop their ICT skills as early as possible.

Kareem's teachers started teaching him to touch-type in Year 4. To begin with he was very slow and frustrated his teachers as he could not produce much work in lessons. After two years, with regular practice, Kareem's typing skills have really improved. He can now communicate in writing much more easily than before and his confidence and self-esteem have soared.

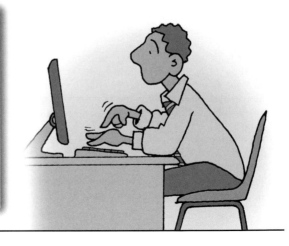

Making use of ICT

Many learners enjoy using a computer, and developing specific ICT skills can be highly motivating for them. Initially, typing will be slow – as with any new skill – but over time, it is likely to improve, unlike their handwriting. ICT can be used to:

- Compensate for poor handwriting - it allows pupil to focus more on content and helps them to organise, restructure and edit work easily
- Access text, graphics or sound to suit the pupil's preferred learning style
- Develop study techniques, such as 'Mind maps'
- Develop reading, spelling and grammar using appropriate specialist software, eg Text Help, spell checkers, grammar checkers and word prediction software

Life skills & self-help skills

Learners with dyspraxia have problems with their independent living skills and some struggle to perform everyday living activities. They may have difficulty following the whole-school timetable, completing homework assignments, maintaining their own personal hygiene, appearance, eating, crossing roads or riding a bus independently.

Pupils may appear slow and disorganised with tasks and may need a structured individual and small-step programme to develop their organisational, self-help and independent skills.

It is important to share your concerns with parents and the individual pupil and prioritise the skills you need to teach first. Discuss the plan and strategies with them, so that they know their personal targets and understand which techniques will improve their independence and organisation. Pupils need a lot of opportunities to practise learned skills before they feel confident at using them in everyday life as independent learners. A 'peer buddy' system can further support learners to develop independence.

Developing a Dyspraxia-friendly Classroom

Learner, environment and task

You don't need to be an expert in dyspraxia to develop a dyspraxia-friendly classroom. Most of the strategies discussed in this book constitute good classroom practice for all children with specific learning difficulties in these areas.

A dyspraxia-friendly classroom doesn't just focus on a pupil's difficulties, it takes into account the interactions between the learner, their environment and the tasks set. This can be visualised as a triangle:

Teachers with an inclusive and holistic classroom ethos, who consider the learner, the task and the environment together in this way, are able to foster a more supportive and friendly environment for learners with dyspraxia.

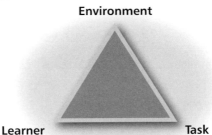

Adapting the learning environment

Like any other learners, pupils with dyspraxia spend a vast amount of time within educational settings. It is important to adjust the learning environment to suit individual needs, so that pupils feel happy, safe, secure, and confident. For a dyspraxia-friendly environment:

- Provide structure and predictability
- Check temperature, light and noise levels in the classroom
- Check furniture layout and height for its suitability
- Create a 'Quiet Corner' or dedicated 'workstation' to carry out certain tasks
- Label equipment, books etc so that they are easy to identify and locate
- Provide a well-organised working area
- Limit the materials/equipment available on the pupil's desk
- Provide opportunities for 'time out' from others, in case the pupil gets too tired or over-excited

Adapting the task

For learners with dyspraxia, the demands of a task need to be flexible, so that they experience success and are able to maintain their confidence and self-esteem. Tasks need to be structured and suitably differentiated.

- Use a problem-solving approach when you set tasks, so pupils can take ownership of their learning
- Explain the purpose of the task and set clear targets/goals
- Review and celebrate their progress with them
- Use other methods than writing to check knowledge and understanding, eg oral presentation
- Prioritise the skills you want to teach and provide opportunities to practise
- Provide materials to aid learning, eg larger print/font, coloured backgrounds, ICT equipment
- Set tasks with minimum writing requirements
- Be realistic about their pace of work and your expectations

Learner's perspectives

It is important to see the pupil as a learner, not just as a 'dyspraxic pupil', and focus on identifying and removing barriers to learning to maximise their potential.

As each pupil with dyspraxia has a different set of difficulties and the degree of severity of each varies, it is unlikely that a single approach will work for all learners. It is vital to understand the individual learner's perspective and their strengths and weaknesses; this can be challenging. For example, some pupils will be able to cope with the demands of reading out loud but others will be too frightened. Similarly, some pupils will be more sensitive than others in coping with environmental noise. Try to:

- Manage your learners' needs by reducing the complexity of tasks and modifying the learning environment
- Understand the learner's point of view and address issues using a problem-solving approach
- Give positive, encouraging feedback whenever possible to develop their confidence, self-esteem and emotional wellbeing
- Make the learner feel enthusiastic about learning new skills and experiencing success
- Liaise with their parents to understand the 'whole pupil'

Transition to secondary school

Any transition is difficult for a pupil with dyspraxia – even the transition from one activity to another or from one classroom to another can be stressful. Moving from primary to secondary school can be particularly challenging and daunting. As the pupil is fully aware of their difficulties, they can experience a lot of anxiety. Careful planning and preparation is required and the plan needs to be shared with the pupil before the move. Here are some useful pointers for successful transition:

- The primary school needs to share information with a key person at the secondary school – this could be a SENCO, inclusion manager or a member of the learning support team. Provide a brief profile of the learner with information on their strengths and weaknesses and effective classroom management strategies

- Discuss the pupil's organisational difficulties with the key person and arrange for extra support, eg in managing class work and homework

- Encourage parents to attend extra meetings with the secondary SENCO/key person at the new school to share relevant details *before* the pupil moves

Transition to secondary school

- Learners with dyspraxia will need to familiarise themselves with the layout of a new school building. The traditional open day visit will not offer enough opportunity for this. Before the pupil moves to their new school, arrange one or more after-school visits, when the building will be less crowded, for better familiarisation of the environment and to meet a key person

- During visits, ask the key person to provide a colour-coded school plan – teaching areas for different subjects could be colour-coded

- Check lunch arrangements/procedures with the new school and teach the pupil, prior to arriving, when to bring lunch money and where to hand it in

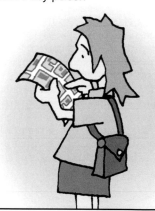

Organising personal belongings

Their poor organisational skills mean that pupils with dyspraxia may find it hard to get to lessons on time, misreading the day and time of lessons and ending up in the wrong one. Organising their books, equipment, homework diary, and so on takes real effort. The struggle to organise themselves and their work makes pupils with dyspraxia feel stressed. You can help them by:

- Providing extra copies of their timetable, colour-coded according to subject. (If you can, match the subject colour with the colour of their exercise books)
- Encouraging them to use a transparent pencil case so they can easily find pens and pencils
- Communicating with parents regularly, so that they can build a routine for checking school bags, homework diary etc
- Teaching them to prioritise their tasks, manage their time and use visual aids such as tick lists to check what is finished and what still needs to be done

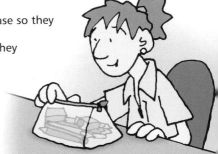

Managing written class work

At secondary school, students are expected to write a lot more than they were at primary, with both speed and accuracy. Students with dyspraxia struggle to keep up with note-taking and writing in general. They may appear to never be ready for work and have problems in starting and/or completing tasks. They may not be able to finish written tasks within a given time in class. Consider the following support strategies:

- Encourage them to use an alternative method of recording, eg dictaphone or computer
- If their keyboard skills are poor, provide extra tuition – this could be extra lessons or software that develops typing skills
- Provide a photocopied worksheet with blank spaces for the pupil to fill in (cloze procedure)
- Use mind maps and concept maps to minimise writing

Remember that pupils with dyspraxia often put in twice as much effort as their peers to produce the same amount of work; as a result they get tired very quickly.

Managing homework

The extra energy that pupils with dyspraxia expend during the school day makes them more tired after school than their peers. Completing and bringing in homework on time can be very challenging and stressful. It can feel overwhelming for pupils and can be a battle for parents.

If there are difficulties completing homework, check the reasons behind this – is the pupil capable of completing the work or do they simply lack motivation? Try to:

- Provide differentiated homework or allow the pupil to complete unfinished class work at home
- Arrange for an adult to write down homework instructions and due dates in the pupil's homework diary, or set the homework well before the end of the lesson allowing plenty of time for the pupil to record it
- Allow extra time for project work – this could be extended over a period of weeks
- Provide a 'buddy' who can check whether the pupil has completed their homework
- Provide a specific area for handing in completed homework

Some final thoughts

It is very easy to misunderstand pupils with dyspraxia as they do not follow a set pattern. Their needs are complex and varied in nature. Their underlying motor skill impairments have a significant impact on many other areas, including their social, emotional, physical and intellectual development. A good understanding of their difficulties is vital in order to identify and address them effectively.

From even a young age, these learners will pick up negative comments about their difficulties. Understanding the nature of these difficulties will help you address their problems in a supportive way. If learners feel supported and understood, they are more likely to be motivated to attempt new tasks.

The right kind of support and encouragement, together with timely interventions enable pupils with dyspraxia to learn and develop coping strategies, although their ability to cope in certain situations varies widely.

Pupils with dyspraxia need to feel confident in order to cope better with the challenges they face at school.

Summary

- Dyspraxia describes the difficulty planning and carrying out motor movements in sequence, in the absence of muscular paralysis or weakness
- Difficulties with movements can significantly impact a learner's social, emotional, behavioural and intellectual development
- Each pupil with dyspraxia will have their own strengths and weaknesses in their learning
- Early identification of a learner's difficulties and appropriate and timely interventions are the key to success
- Pupils need to develop self-esteem and confidence alongside their learning
- A good understanding and knowledge of dyspraxia is vital for every school; a positive attitude from teachers can make as much difference as interventions
- A co-ordinated approach from different professionals is important in addressing the diverse needs of pupils with dyspraxia
- General 'good practice' classroom strategies are useful for pupils who are mildly affected by dyspraxia, who may never be formally identified
- Pupils with dyspraxia will never 'grow out' of their condition but with the right kind of interventions they can be successful learners

Further reading

Creating Circles of Friends
by D. Wilson and C. Newton
Published by Inclusive Solutions, 2003

Developmental Co-ordination Disorder
by M.F. Ball
Published by Jessica Kingsley, 2002

**Developmental Dyspraxia, Identification
and Intervention – A Manual for Parents
and Professionals**
by M. Portwood
Published by David Fulton, 2006

**Dyspraxia/Developmental Co-ordination
Disorder**
by A. Kirby
Published by Souvenir Press Ltd, 2011

Focus on Dyspraxia: Lets Move On
by C. Macintyre
Published by NASEN, 2003

Helping Children with Dyspraxia
by M. Boon
Published by Jessica Kingsley, 2002

**How to Understand and Support Children
with Dyspraxia**
by L. Addy
Published by LDA, 2004

**Inclusion for Children with Dyspraxia/DCD
– A Handbook for Teachers**
by K. Ripley
Published by David Fulton, 2003

**Recognising Developmental Co-ordination
disorders: Developmental Dyspraxia
Explained**
Published by Dyspraxia Foundation, 1998

Resources, websites, handwriting programmes

Inclusive Technology
Riverside Court, Huddersfield Road,
Oldham, OL3 5FZ.
Tel: 01457 819790
www.inclusive.co.uk

Crick Software Ltd
Crick House, Boarden Close,
Moulton Park, Northampton, NN3 6LF
Tel: 01604 671691
www.cricksoft.com – for Clicker 4 & 5

www.dyslexic.com – literacy and numeracy,
mind-mapping and note-taking software
www.spark-space.com – software for essay
writing and spelling
www.widgit.com – first keys to literacy
www.boxofideas.org – search on 'dyspraxia'

The Speed-Up! – A kinaesthetic
programme to develop fluent handwriting.
L. Addy, LDA Publications, 2004

Start Write, Stay Right – A whole child
approach to handwriting
A. Harris & J. Taylor, TTS Group Ltd, 2007

Write-Dance – A music and movement
programme to develop pre-writing and
writing skills.
R. Oussoren, Lucky Duck Publications, 2000

Write from the Start – Developing the
fine-motor and perceptual skills for
effective handwriting.
I. Teodorescu, & L. Addy, LDA Publications,
1996

Suppliers and equipment

Sloping boards, reading rulers, special pens, pencil grips, etc.
www.backinaction.co.uk – portable writing slopes, seat wedges
www.beesneez.co.uk – sloping boards
www.cambridgehouse-dyslexia.co.uk – pencil grips, Stabilo S' Move Easy Handwriting Pen, coloured overlays and eye level reading rulers
www.crossboweducation.co.uk – tinted exercise books, sand timers, memory booster games
www.hope-education.co.uk
www.ldalearning.com
www.posturite.co.uk – seat wedges, speech recognition software, eg Dragon Naturally Speaking
www.taskmasteronline.co.uk
www.yoropen.pen – for the Yoro pen and Yoro pencil

Touch-typing programmes
www.sense-lang.org/typing
www.bbc.co.uk/schools/typing

Touch-type Read and Spell – systematic typing course based on the Alpha to Omega reading and spelling programme for primary and secondary schools. Centres throughout the UK. Tel 020 8464 1330

Useful contacts

Dyspraxia Foundation
8 West Alley, Hitchin, Hertfordshire SG5 1EG
Tel: 01462 455016
www.dyspraxiafoundation.org.uk
Provides support and resource materials for adults and children with dyspraxia.

The Dyscovery Centre
Felthorpe House, Caerleon Campus, Lodge Road, Caerleon, Newport NP18 3QR
Tel: 01633 432330
The centre assesses and treats children and adults with learning difficulties including dyspraxia. It also provides resources and equipment.

The National Association of Special Educational Needs (NASEN)
NASEN House, Amber Business Village, Amber Close, Amington, Tamworth, Staffs B77 4RP
Tel: 01827 311500
www.nasen.org.uk

About the author

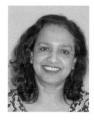

Afroza Talukdar BSc. (Hons), MSc., PGCE, MEd., PGCert. (Dyspraxia)

Afroza Talukdar qualified as a secondary science teacher over 20 years ago and has taught in mainstream primary and secondary schools. Currently, and for the past 15 years, she has been working as SEN advisory teacher for a local authority, providing specialist advice on SEN issues to both primary and secondary school teachers as well as running courses, training sessions and organising conferences. Over the years, she has developed a specialist interest in dyspraxia, working as a specialist teacher providing advice to mainstream teachers on how best to address the needs of children with motor co-ordination difficulties. Afroza has completed a number of postgraduate qualifications reflecting her increasing specialisation in the field of SEN and dyspraxia.

Afroza is a member of the education panel on the Dyspraxia Foundation. She has a national publication on provision and assessment maps on dyspraxia, aimed at improving provision for pupils with dyspraxia in a mainstream classroom setting.

Afroza's vast experience working with pupils with dyspraxia, their teachers and their parents has provided unique insight and understanding and has inspired her to write this book. She can be contacted at: afrozatalukdar@gmail.com

Order form

Your details

Name _____

Position _____

School _____

Address _____

_____

_____

Telephone _____

Fax _____

E-mail _____

VAT No. (EC only) _____

Your Order Ref _____

Please send me:

No.
copies

Dyspraxia/DCD _____ Pocketbook [ ]

_____ Pocketbook [ ]

_____ Pocketbook [ ]

_____ Pocketbook [ ]

Order by Post
Teachers' Pocketbooks
Laurel House, Station Approach
Alresford, Hants. SO24 9JH UK

Order by Phone, Fax or Internet
Telephone: +44 (0)1962 735573
Facsimile: +44 (0)1962 733637
Email: sales@teacherspocketbooks.co.uk
Web: www.teacherspocketbooks.co.uk

Customers in USA should contact:
2427 Bond Street, University Park, IL 60466
Tel: 866 620 6944   Facsimile: 708 534 7803
Email: mp.orders@ware-pak.com
Web: www.teacherspocketbooks.com